Climate Change

How Fast Are We Changing Our Planet?

I0420736

By

Fhilcar Faunillan

Fhilcar Faunillan

Climate Change

The information provided herein is stated to be truthful and consistent, in that any liability, in terms of inattention or otherwise, by any usage or abuse of any policies, processes, or directions contained within is the solitary and utter responsibility of the recipient reader. Under no circumstances will any legal responsibility or blame be held against the publisher for any reparation, damages, or monetary loss due to the information herein, either directly or indirectly.

Respective authors own all copyrights not held by the publisher.

The information herein is offered for informational purposes solely, and is universal as so. The presentation of the information is without contract or any type of guarantee assurance.

The trademarks that are used are without any consent, and the publication of the trademark is without permission or backing by the trademark owner. All trademarks and brands within this book are for clarifying purposes only and are the owned by the owners themselves, not affiliated with this document.

Table of Contents

INTRODUCTION

I want to thank you and congratulate you for downloading the book, *"Climate Change: How Fast Are We Changing Our Planet?"*.

Nowadays, we get off on anything that is fast and all its synonyms – fast food, quick service, fast delivery, etc. Take more than a week for your ordered product to be shipped and you blow a gasket. Mornings are blurred memories full of instant noodles and easy to prepare cereals. We hurry through life by pressing down on the accelerator of our cars so we can race with others to get to our destinations. But in every squeeze of insecticide cans to kill off cockroaches or in every flick of the switch to turn the lights on, we – unwittingly for some, indifferently for others – are affecting our planet in a way that is, more often than not, destructive. We are changing our planet and we are changing it fast. How fast, you may ask? Fast enough that efforts to curb the significantly detrimental effects of human activities would not be sufficient in the long run.

Blame being busy or simple self-centeredness but we hardly notice what is going on in our environment. Blame our sense of entitlement and superiority or some other human quality but simply put, we do not care about it. We think that nature is for our taking, that we can do with it whatever we want. We throw garbage everywhere even if there is obviously a huge sign right in front us discouraging the act.

I am pretty sure you have went through this phase. Perhaps, you are *stuck* at this phase but I remember when I was a child and I did not really give a damn about throwing my candy wrappers and junk food containers on the street once they are empty of food. It took a scolding from my parents and school lessons to make me stop doing it. But for some people, no amount of knowledge and reprimands could change one's attitude towards environmental preservation. And here stems most of the issues we are facing as of today in regards to our world.

Before you dive into this book, here is a food for thought: there is no disconnection between what we do and what our planet feels because of it. So, here is a little exercise for you. Think of an activity – any human activity – that you feel do not have any negative effect on the environment. Cooking? Showering? Reading? You choose. And keep your answer in mind and as you go through this book, find out if your answer is correct. If you are wrong, learn just in what way human activities could impact the world.

Speaking of, one of the most notable bearing human activities have on our planet is climate change. This is pretty much a familiar term. I would even bet a thousand bucks that you are living under a rock if you have not heard a thing or two about climate change. In this book, not only will climate change will be tackled but also other human activities that have drastically affected our planet and prodded it to change for the worse. I am going to talk about the earth bombs that we have individually wielded and detonated to destroy our Mother Earth.

Thanks again for downloading this book, I hope you enjoy it!

Chapter 1 - Plants vs. Humans

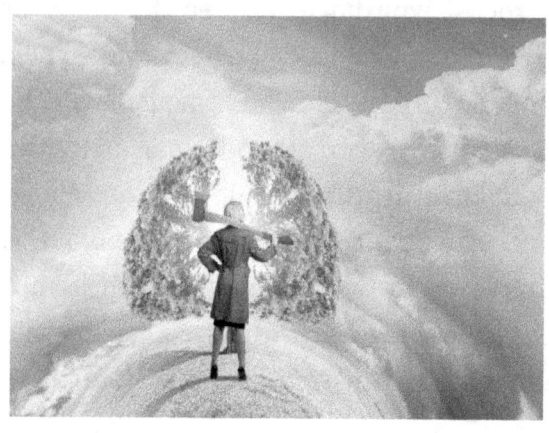

It can be argued that human progress, specifically technological advancement, does not come hand in hand with environmental sustainability. Various environmentalists have pushed that these two concepts have an inverse relationship with each other. The more technology develops, the poorer the quality of the environment. Though it is not entirely true, this argument does have a point. At first glance, you can observe how

Climate Change

depleted a forest becomes due to construction projects and establishment of industries. Miles and miles of wildlife are cleared out so there can be space for subdivisions. Every year, more and more trees are cut down for various reasons and rivers are drained to serve some industrial purpose.

Take a look around you and perhaps look back to five or 10 years ago. What changed in your neighborhood? Were there still trees around or were you born in a gray, cemented city?

There are some of us who still had the pleasure of experiencing climbing up the trees when we were still children and bathing in the river. I was one of those blessed with the opportunity to live a life in a place where chirping crickets are heard when it is getting dark and where I sort of had to risk myself a little to be able to reach fruits high up in the trees so I could munch on something as I play around my grandparents' farm. When I went to the city to study, it was a huge shock to find smoke being blasted on my face without any warning, to be in the middle of rushing people seemingly desperate to get where they want to go, and to settle with junk food for my snacks. But you get used to it. And I guess there is where another of our faults is. We get used to things. When trees are being chopped down and grasses are cleared so that a condominium or commercial building could be built upon the land, we feel the loss of the shade and fresh air at first but then, we get used to the feeling of suffocating heat. We get used to news of flashfloods. We get used to typhoon warnings. We get used to natural calamities. We think that there is no other choice but get adapted to what is happening around us today because in the first place, what can you do? You can't stop a whole village from being destroyed by a storm surge. It is out of your hands.

Climate Change

However, what we fail to acknowledge is the fact that whatever natural catastrophe might happen probably came into being because of our actions. Flash floods happened because we cut down trees and we got used to large-scale deforestation. We got used to environmental policies not being implemented and followed by the constituents. We got used to not finding a link between our actions and the state of our environment.

But one thing is for sure and people need to bear this in mind: *almost every anthropogenic move has an impact on the environment.* When you cook eggs every morning or take a shower, you are leaving a footprint that further damages nature. Nope. It is not a visible footprint in the sand but one that, when combined with other people's footprints, contribute to Earth's destruction and produces palpable environmental issues. This is what we call *carbon footprint.*

Every person, organization, or even as simple as an action leaves a carbon footprint which refers to the total amount of greenhouse gas or GHG emitted. Every car that you see has a corresponding set of carbon footprint. Even farming and fishing has a carbon footprint. Almost every action nowadays emit GHG because processes and results require the emission of it. Take cooking for example. Let us not compute the carbon footprint gained from the production of bacon and focus on just cooking it. To satisfy your stomach with the smell and taste of bacon, you need to cook it on your electric stove using oil. The harnessing, production, and distribution of electricity emits GHG and same applies to oil. And as you burn your bacon into a crisp, you release gases into the atmosphere.

You might think that a mundane thing such as taking a shower can hardly affect the environment but here is where you are wrong. Even eating meat instead of vegetables do. In fact, those who are meat-eaters have a larger amount of carbon footprint compared to vegetarians.

What I have touched so far demonstrates how humans have the capability of denting the defenses of Mother Earth. In the next chapter, I am going into details of the major human activity that has changed the planet into what it is right now and how their effects branch out to produce multitudes of concerns including ecological, geographical, and anthropological.

Chapter 2 - Changing the Planet, One Human Evil Deed at a Time

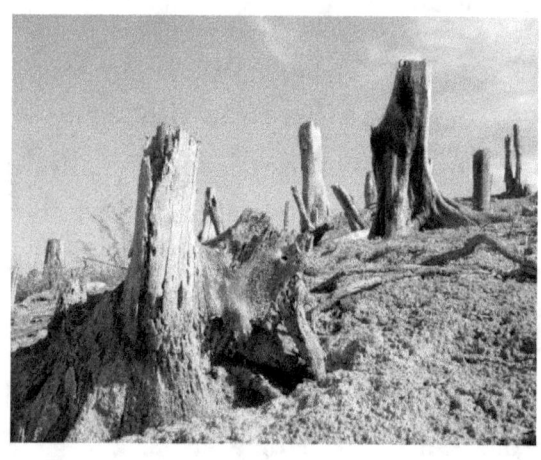

It has been thousands of years since the first humans have occupied this planet. Early human beings started with hunting and gathering – professions that are heavily dependent on resources they could wrestle out from the environment. As population grew, there was a change in needs and the nomadic lifestyle they embraced could no longer be ideal so humans settled in and tilled the land to grow food for their communities. Then, they developed tools in order to make life easier.

And now, here we are in the 21st century, all settled in our homes and surrounded by all forms of technology. This time around, we hardly ever think about where we got the stuff we think we can't live without. How did a mobile phone come to be? What were the raw materials used? Was our natural resources drained in order to create this tiny box of radiation that we use every day to amuse ourselves?

From the very first attempt to fulfill human needs and further progress, we have affected nature. And all throughout history, there were major human activities that were developed in order to satisfy our goals (e.g. have more food, build a shelter). And these activities are still being practiced today and are continually changing our planet.

1. Deforestation

Cutting down of trees and massive deforestation efforts throughout the centuries have proven to be damaging not only to the environment but their effects also rebound back to humans. Ever since the agricultural revolution where people shifted from their nomadic lifestyle in order to settle in one locale, cutting of trees have been practiced in order to clear out lands for the cultivation of plants and domestication of animals. This cultural change has led to more food supply that was stable but it decreased the quality of the environment.

Deforestation happens for various reasons, most of which benefit humans. To begin with, trees are cut down in order to provide fuel. Forests are cleared in order to pave way for the construction of settlements and to serve as pasture for livestock animals. In some cases, deforestation was used as a strategy in wars to rob enemies of resources and cover.

It can occur naturally but the upsetting fact is that major cases have been human-induced. In many countries, deforestation is still an ongoing issue and the large-scale exhibition of it can be attributed to not just individual human behavior but also to a lack of environmental laws and strict policy implementations.

This phenomenon has resulted in numerous environmental tragedies including desertification, displacement of populations, biodiversity loss, species extinction, and changes to climatic conditions.

Deforestation also has an atmospheric impact and affects both the geography and the climate. Most important to note is how it contributes to global warming and how it does not help alleviate the issue of the presence of greenhouse gases in the atmosphere. Without plants and trees to process it, carbon dioxide remains stagnant in the atmosphere. During photosynthesis, plants process out the carbon present in CO_2 from the atmosphere, stores it in plant tissues, and releases oxygen as a by-product. But it takes a large amassing of plants and trees for a significant amount of carbon to be taken up. Cutting down hundreds of them is ultimately a bad move at the end of the day. Furthermore, the burning of trees paves the way for the stored carbon in the plant tissues to be released back to the atmosphere.

Moreover, deforestation similarly has an unwanted and undesirable say on the water cycle. Trees extract water from the ground and makes it available for taking by the land and the atmosphere. Without trees to transpire water, a drier climate would be the result.

Furthermore, soil erosion becomes more pronounced when forest cover is minimized since the land's ability to intercept and retain rainwater is decreased. So, instead of locking in precipitation so it could seep into groundwater systems, they run off. In severe cases of downpour, this water runoff could translate into flash flooding. The topmost layers of the land which favors growth because of the amount of nutrients in them have been eroded.

2. Urbanization

Simply put, urbanization, the way we do it right now, is good for humans and bad for the environment. Well, it is not a crime to want to build houses and infrastructures for human utilization but we lack the ability of taking the state of our environment into consideration as we build buildings over lands that used to house ecological organisms.

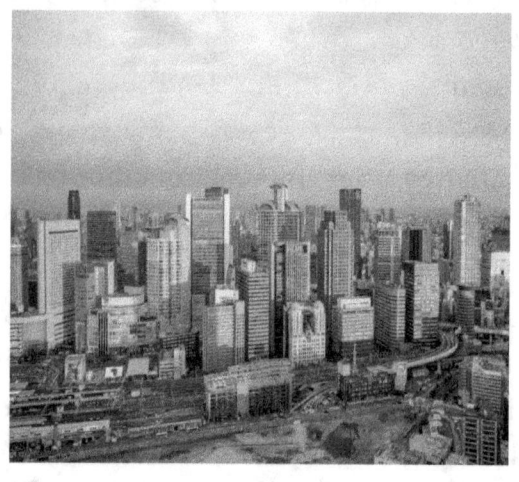

Builders decide to wipe out ecosystems involving a multitude of organisms to create homes, shopping centers, schools, and businesses, displacing animals and destroying plant life. And it just does not stop there. As years pass by, humans expand their properties to construct roads and more communities.

At the end of the day, there is a conflict between environmental preservation and human development. Most of us find it easy to pick a side. Of course we would push for human development in order to survive. Only a small percentage of our population realizes that there can be a balance between the two.

3. Farming and irrigation

Hand in hand with the growth in human population is the need for agricultural land expansion in order to supply sufficient food. The problem is, though in order to facilitate farming, people are turning to deforestation in order to clear out forests and grow crops. As already discussed in the previous item, deforestation takes a very great toll on the environment.

Moreover, the fertilizers that farmers use to grow their crops have proven to be detrimental to various ecosystems. Some of these fertilizers put human health at risk and fertilizer runoff from farmlands which are usually carried into bodies of water are killing marine organisms.

In addition, irrigation, which involves the drawing out of water from a water source such as groundwater, lake or river, and distributing it over a targeted area, is another problem. Irrigation is very much useful in farming because it makes it possible for crops and plants to become watered.

As much as it helps agriculture, irrigation provides adverse impacts on the environment. If the system is drawing out water from rivers, it could reduce the river's downstream flow and this would lead to loss of vital wetlands, diminished amount of drinking water for households and industries, reduced opportunities for fishing, and lesser discharge of water into the sea.

4. Greenhouse gas emissions

One of the most pressing issues of today (i.e. global warming) has been mainly attributed to human-induced greenhouse gas emissions. Yes, it is true that the planet's climate has changed numerous times throughout history but scientist have concluded that the rise in temperature we experience today cannot be accounted for by natural variability. This means that the only explanation for the rapid warming is wide-spread human activity, particularly the emission of carbon dioxide or CO2 and other greenhouse gases.

From what we have learned from our science classes, a modicum amount of greenhouse gases is important for life to survive on Earth. The greenhouse effect is a natural and necessary warming process. Carbon dioxide and other GHG which are always present in the Earth's atmosphere serve to trap heat, warming the planet, encouraging growth, and keeping us from being frozen to death. However, the natural greenhouse effect is being strengthened by human activities like burning of fuels to the point that it is rising the global temperature.

GHG can be released through a lot of media. Production, distribution, and consumption of fuel, food, manufactured goods, services, and infrastructures as well as transport are just some of the ways that people discharge GHG.

It has been reported that concentrations of man-made greenhouse gases have exploded ever since the Industrial revolution. This is understandable since that period marked the invention of a lot of machines (e.g. steam engine) that burn fuels and releases GHG in the process. Concentration of three major greenhouse gases, to be specific, continue to rise every year namely carbon dioxide, methane, and nitrous oxide.

GHG emissions is a serious concern because of the consequences. The warming of the planet has now led to major events that are legitimately causes of concern. Sea levels are rising, glaciers and ice sheets are melting, typhoons have become stronger, and heat waves have been more extreme. If we do not rein in when it comes to pumping greenhouse gases into the atmosphere, the state of the environment would just worsen in the decades to come.

5. Coal mining and burning

Diverse is the consequence of coal mining and burning. Some of the issues linked to it include water and air pollution, land transformation, and waste management.

Strip mining, in particular, changes the landscape of the place being mined, reducing the quality of the natural environment. Moreover, mining in a particular site displaces human settlements and animals who might be calling the place their home. Aside from damaging wildlife, strip mining also harms the genetic profile of the soil and can make the land unusable in the future as it eliminates the nutrients of the soil that makes it fit for vegetation.

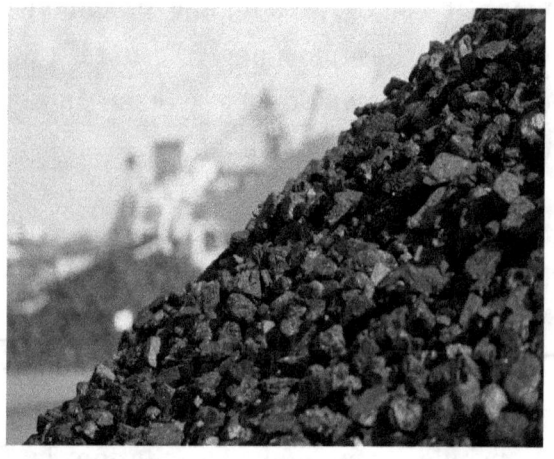

Mining, as it strips off the vegetative cover of the soil and removes the topmost layers, increases the amount of dust around the mining location. The higher quantity in the mining operation lowers the air quality around it and affects the growth capacity of the surrounding areas. Workers and humans near the location could also suffer health problems because of it.

As for the burning of coal, it is actually the largest contributor to the man-made greenhouse gases in the atmosphere. Not only does it releases carbon dioxide, mining of coal also produces methane which is a potent GHG.

6. Meat production

Even meat production has an adverse outcome on the environment. Associated with the production and distribution of meat for human consumption are damages on the environment because of the utilization of fossil energy, land resources, and water. Greenhouse gases are also emitted in the processes involved in the production. And since human beings are not really picky and could target almost any edible animal, species endangerment is also one of the negative effects of this human activity.

7. Mining

If protective measures are not prepared and observed, the negative effects of mining can be extremely environmentally harsh. First off, mining contributes to water pollution because of runoff. High concentrations of toxic chemicals like mercury, arsenic, and sulfuric acid can devastate plant, human, and animal life. Even the runoff of non-toxic soil debris can stunt the vegetation of surrounding places.

Biodiversity will also be touched when there is mining in an area formerly rich with life. The main mine-related cause for diversity loss would be the eradication of the habitat of organisms but what can also kill off animals, microorganisms, and vegetal are the toxic minerals extracted from the materials mined. The most vulnerable here are endemics species because their survival is highly dependent on a certain set of environmental conditions. Even a slight shift or change in their habitat could put them in jeopardy.

8. Transportation

The environmental impacts of transport should be seriously noted because it is a heavy user of energy and needs a great quantity of petroleum whose burning contributes to the increasing concentration of greenhouse gases in the atmosphere.

Every day, roads are getting more crowded because more and more people purchase cars. And for every car that means a higher quantity of emitted carbon dioxide. This makes transport the fastest-growing sector when it comes to emission quantities and is therefore a very expansive contributor to global warming. In some countries, emissions of individual vehicles have been controlled but what progress these regulations have made were offset by the growing number of cars.

Because of the quantity of vehicles on the road, traffic congestion is a common problem and automobile-oriented urban sprawls have been pushed in order to accommodate them. Habitats and lands are then cleared in order to expand roads and create more paths.

9. Plastic production

The advancement in technology has paved the way for the development of new materials. One of the most notable inventions in history is plastic, a material that like most of the stuff nowadays contain chemical components that could remain in the environment for thousands of years without decomposing and could have long-lasting effects on planetary cycles.

Industries annually produce billions and billions of tons of plastics and they remain in the planet because they do not rot. Imagine just how much plastic there is right now ever since they were invented. Have you heard of an island of plastic floating somewhere in one of the major oceans of the world? Yep. That was a legit news. Actually, it was estimated that there are pieces of plastic for every square mile of ocean.

Plastics, in high concentrations, can disturb animal endocrine systems and cause cancers in some organisms. And not to mention that manufacturing plastics add additional and unwanted GHG in the atmosphere.

Chapter 3 - Climate Change is NOT a Good Change

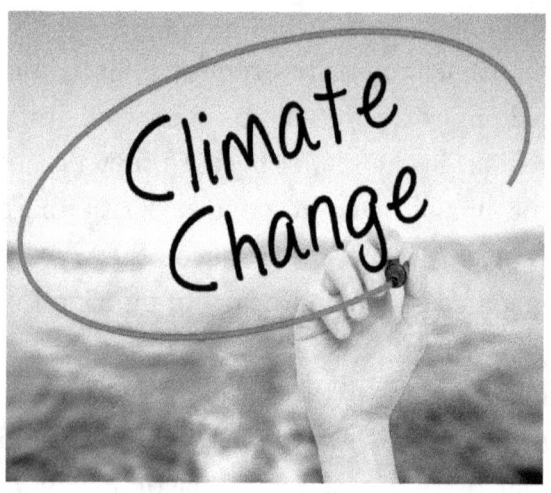

Climate refers to the projected weather condition at a certain place over a period of time. Some places in Japan, for example, will experience winter for a number of weeks while New York City experiences hot days for months. Usually, climate is measured using statistics such as average number of rainy days, mean temperature, among others. Case in point, in Africa, there is a predicted frequency of droughts in certain regions. Cities or countries can have a set climate statistics.

When we say *climate change*, it denotes that over the years, the aforementioned statistics have altered. Climate change is not such an alarming issue as it is a normal phenomenon if not for the fact that our climate is changing too fast. In fact, scientists believed that the change we are experiencing right now is one of the largest climatic changes ever since the extinction of the dinosaurs. And what demanded researchers to understand its causes and the impacts it would have to our planet – for humans, animals, and plants – is the pace of the change. Compared to the climate changes in the previous 65 million years, the one we have right now is at the minimum ten times quicker.

At the rate we are going on right now, it would take only a few more decades for the planet to become an unsafe space to live in for human beings, animals, and plants. In the near future, we will be overwhelmed with typhoons, killer heat waves, flashfloods, and droughts. Coastal villages will be wiped out if not by storm surges then by the rising sea level. Too many human activities (e.g. mindless consumption, technology, economic growth) are just in play and are succeeding in destabilizing the planet.

Climate change happens because of two reasons: natural causes and human-related causes. As mentioned, climate change is a given part of Earth's dynamics. Interactions amongst the different elements present on Earth contribute to a natural change in climate statistics. Temperature during the Ice Age is definitely different compared to the average temperature of today. Usually, the common driving forces behind the change in climate include the radiation from the sun, movement of the planetary orbit and axis, and alterations in the composition of gas in the atmosphere. Natural events such as volcanic eruptions can also be a factor.

Yet, what hastens climate change are pressures that are mostly the responsibility of humans. A significant number of scientists concur that what is to be blamed for global warming, in particular, is anthropogenic activity which is extensively widespread. This century has seen a significant increase in global temperature and it is very probable that the cause of that, not taking into consideration the other substantial and damaging human activities at this point, is the gas emissions that we are responsible for. During the past century, researchers insist that it is highly unlikely that the global rise in temperature that we have been experiencing is mainly due to natural causes alone because the warming occurred at times when natural driving forces would have produced cooling both in the ocean and the atmosphere instead of the opposite.

Ultimately, the effects of climate change will touch different countries – developed or not – various ecosystems, and numerous economies, among others. Nature will not play favorite. And the survival of human beings will depend on both these systems vulnerability to climate change and their capability of adapting to a changing world.

History have proven that human societies and ecosystems are resilient and possess the admirable ability of responding to threats and adapting to different conditions. The question is, with the severity of the impending climate change, will the organisms of the planet still learn to survive? Unlike the other climate changes in previous millions of years, the one that we are facing today is human-induced and it may demand another set of approaches in order to battle it and ensure the continued existence of the natural environment and of the human society. In line with this, along with shedding a light on the science behind climate change, research has also made it a point to learn what actions can be taken in order to limit the effect of climate change.

Chapter 4 - Climate Change Consequences

These were just part of theories before but what scientists have predicted to be the impacts of climate change and global warming are now translated into reality. The second half of this century have seen extreme storms that killed thousands of people, flashfloods out of nowhere, and other life-threatening natural calamities. In this chapter, I will go over several of the natural events associated with climate change that we are experiencing today.

1. Rising sea level

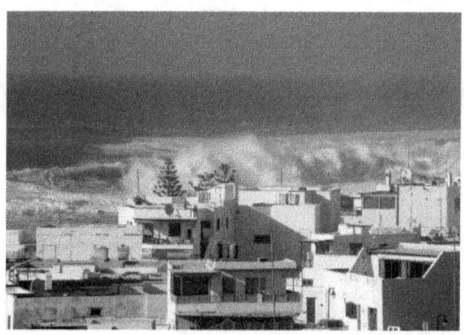

Climate Change

A rise in sea level is brought about by the melting of glaciers and ice sheets in the world and the warming of oceans which leads to the thermal expansion of seas. This is one of the most serious and disastrous effects of global warming. It is expected that by the end of this century, sea level may increase to a couple of feet higher than it is today if the emission of greenhouse gases is not reined in.

Rising sea level is especially catastrophic because of its severe impact in plant, animal, and human life. Edges of forests near coasts have and will drown. And alarmingly, mangrove forests that serve as habitat for important marine species (e.g. fish, shrimps) and birds will also been flooded. These forests also aid in protecting coasts from waves and storm surges and without them, there is no buffer that could prevent water from affecting man-made coastal settlements.

Coastal communities that are low-lying all over the world will be inundated. Just in the US, around half of the population resides close to the ocean. Archipelagic countries and those near major bodies of water are also at risk of being swamped. For underdeveloped nations without strong physical barriers such as manmade seawalls, millions of people can end up getting displaced by even a moderate rise in sea level as it will submerge islands and coastal areas.

More than that, rising of seal level could also contaminate water sources especially groundwater supply and fresh surface water with salty water. The problem would then cross to include problems regarding health and supply of basic necessities.

In addition, as hard as it is to stabilize the rise of our atmospheric temperature, it is even more difficult to address the issue of rising sea level. And this is why it is an imperative for people to put the brakes on emitting greenhouse gas.

2. Torrential rains and flooding

The second half of this century has experienced a significant increase in the frequency and intensity of rain. This is one of the pieces of evidence of global warming as higher temperatures lead to faster evaporation and more water vapor in the air, making downpours heavier. As a result of heavier rainfall, risks of flooding has also heightened.

In some countries, accounts of heavy rainfall included stories of landslides and flooding that killed thousands of people (e.g. Venezuela in 1999). The thing about rainfalls caused by global warming is that they are not only extreme but are also abnormal because they happen outside of the set rainy season of a location. At times, they are not even brought about by tropical cyclones or hurricanes.

El Niño is not helping either. A phase where waters in the eastern Pacific is warmer than average and tropical trade winds weaker than average, El Niño events have become more frequent and intense. Usually, they last around a year and happen once every 2 to 7 years but recent decades have seen more long-lasting El Niño.

One might wonder what El Niño has to do with rains and flooding and with global warming. As the planet warms, El Niño will become more intense and the resulting temperature would facilitate the occurrence of both droughts and floods.

3. Droughts

Paradoxically, with an increase chances of more flooding events comes a higher likelihood as well of severe and frequent droughts. If the temperature rises, the rate of evaporation is faster and this takes the moisture out of the soil and bodies of water. If precipitation does not ensue fast enough to replenish, lands will become drier.

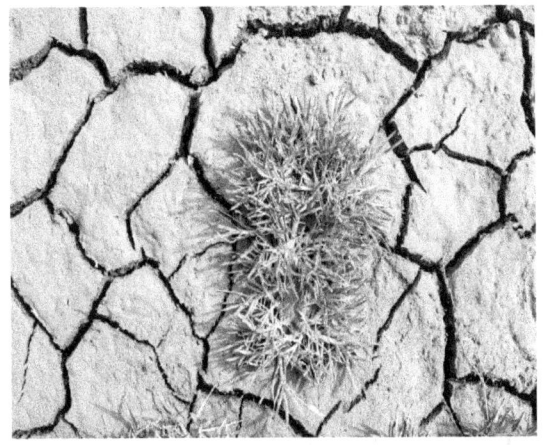

When the soil is dry, solar energy is not used up to evaporate water since there is no moisture left to absorb. Instead, energy is relegated to heightening the temperature of the soil and the air around it and leaves the land more parched.

Plants die and the soil becomes inhospitable for growing things especially when sources of water are also affected and there is no other way to wet the ground.

And it could be difficult to get out of the drought for dry lands will create a cycle. Because moisture in the soil is depleted, there is less evaporation in the air and this would mean the atmosphere can't enable precipitation. At the end of the day, soils will become drier.

4. Wildfires

Global warming is also expected to play a part in more instances of wildfire. As previously mentioned, droughts can become a given and the burning heat of the land and the lack of rainfall is a good combination for fires to develop.

To add, a rise in temperature will instigate outbreak of insects that eat wood, killing trees and turning them into dry fuel that will assist creation of forest fires.

5. Changes in weather patterns

There used to be an expected pattern when it comes to weather in different places. The countries near the Pacific Ocean, for example, can expect a certain number of storms to come annually. But, weather patterns are now changing. Instead of the usual moderate typhoons, out of nowhere, more powerful and damaging storms bulldoze communities and kill lives. In recent years, weather events have become more intense.

6. Super typhoons and hurricanes

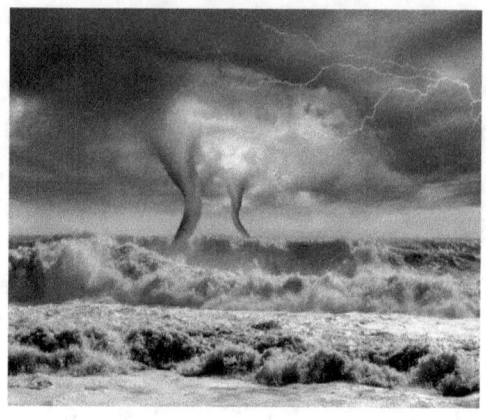

This decade have seen super typhoons and it raised the question regarding the probable connection between climate change and hurricanes. Now, it has become clearer to scientists that there *is*. Hurricanes in all oceans are now stronger due to the state of the oceans. As hurricanes pull their strength from the temperature of ocean surface waters, the rise in temperature have made hurricanes more intense. As both hydrological and atmospheric aspects of the planet continue to heat in the future, we can expect more devastating typhoons to come.

Chapter 5 - Socio-Economic Impact of Climate Change

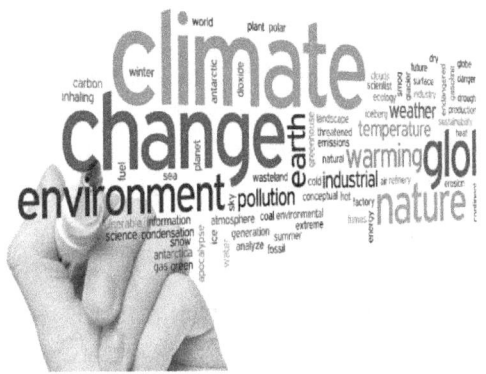

There is a reason why human activities that are now damaging the planet and are bringing about climate change are considered bombs. When they go off, no one is spared. Animals, plants, humans – all of them will be affected. And this is why scientists are working hard to spread the word about climate change, in the hopes that each one of us will do our part in responding to it in one way or another. Because the truth is, climate change and all its associated natural calamities will kill people and will change their lives the way we changed the planet.

The most obvious socio-economic impact of climate change pertains to the health and wellbeing of human beings. Mortality will be greatly disadvantaged once disasters strike.

1. General health

There are certain populations who are more at risk of experiencing the adverse health impacts of a changing climate and these include those who are very young, elderly, living alone, poor, and disabled. People who also have existing serious medical problems could become vulnerable. In addition, people living in vulnerable urban neighborhoods that are already strained with inadequate facilities, unreliable infrastructures, and pressing environmental problems are at a disadvantage.

2. Physical health and injuries

Of course, this is influenced by how equipped and prepared a community is but a consequence of the physical processes involved in climate change is loss of life. The news will tell you that significant number of people have died because of storms. The super typhoon that struck the Philippines in 2013, specifically the storm surge that happened, claimed hundreds of lives. Injuries are sustained when houses are flooded and blown away by strong winds.

Climate change, in addition, can have direct and indirect effects on human health. For example, in cases of extreme temperatures, direct effects would include heat strokes and skin problems. Indirect consequences such as the spread of infectious diseases could also prove to be no less fatal to human mortality.

To add, with the rise in global temperature, it is feared that numerous infectious diseases are going to spread. The behavior of disease vectors such as rodents and mosquitoes are affected by moisture and temperature. And in a lot of ways, global warming could prod the increase of vector-borne diseases through a lot of ways. For one, not only can higher temperatures hasten the maturation of specific disease-causing agents but could also lengthen the period during which these agents are active in spreading diseases. Not to mention that the increase in the frequency of heavy rainfall and flooding which are expected to happen in association with global warming will encourage the growth of disease vectors like rats that carry viruses.

3. Psychological health

Mental health could heavily become strained as well as a consequence of climate change. For places who have been and are expected to be hit with natural calamities, anxiety could take a toll on the populace's health. Even responses to climate change such as mitigation and adaptation can provide additional stress. Migrating, for example, from the house you have lived in all your life to a communal residence as preventive measures against an incoming storm could possibly lead to some mental problems.

4. Safety and crime

In times of calamities, disorder within a society is another thing to expect especially if the affected community has yet to see emergency relief and aid from their government. Desperation for the basic necessity such as food, water, and shelter could lead victims to loot and riot. People are aware that the blame for natural disasters does not lie on the shoulders of government officials. However, once it becomes clear that preventive measures and disaster preparedness was inadequate in the part of the government, this is where social unrest comes in.

Goods and services and the delivery of them will also be affected in times of storms, floods, and other natural disasters.

1. Water

Water shortage can become a problem particularly when there is drought. The absence of precipitation can both affect plant growth and human life. The rise of sea level can also lead to freshwater supply getting contaminate by saltwater.

In this case, you would have to treat your water to make it potable.

2. Food

Food and food supplies can be threatened by the stress brought about by climate change. Farming, a major food-producing activity, may not respond well to the brunt of climate change. Even though an increase in the amount of carbon dioxide in the atmosphere could prove instrumental for the growing of plants, it does not always mean there will be more food. Yes, there is a noteworthy amount of CO_2 but along with other greenhouse gases, it will warm temperature and this will damage the crops and the soil they are planted into.

Of course, the effect of climate change on agriculture will depend on crop type, amount of CO_2 in the atmosphere, and level of temperature, among others. For some areas, moderate warning will favor crop growth and pasture lands but in other regions, it could decrease the yields.

3. Land

Cost would have to be shouldered in order to prepare the lands and prevent flooding.

4. Energy

Energy lines will be down and electricity will be disrupted in times of calamities especially during storms. The loss of energy will become devastating and cumbersome for today's society who can hardly function without it. Businesses will be forced to stop manufacturing and distribution of their products. People who are not prepared for disasters will be left in the dark, unable to cook their food or heat their waters.

5. Housing

Millions of people have lost their homes to natural calamities. As scientists predict that more of the disasters associated with climate change are going to ensue in the future, the number of people who will end up homeless will just increase.

Buildings and properties could be lost to floods and typhoons. And it will take additional cost for housing to be reinforced to survive strong winds and rushing waters.

6. Education

Classes will be suspended in cases of storms damaging schools and education buildings. Loss of teaching days can disadvantage students as they will be deprived of enough days to cover their curriculum. Loss of energy could also disable some of the students dependent on electricity to research materials for their classes from fulfilling case works.

7. Employment

Farmers are some of those whose job will be greatly affected with climate change. Droughts can lead to their crops dying, rendering them unable to get any yield. Floods, on the other hand, would still make their business fail because of drowned plants.

One way or another, other businesses will also be disrupted when there are calamities. For examples, raw materials for a company's product could have been destroyed and so they end up with nothing to sell to their customers.

8. Leisure

When you are in the middle of a 2012 film, there is hardly any time to think about recreation and leisure. Calamities could also destroy facilities that provide entertainment to the masses. Historical and cultural landscapes that were once tourist spots could turn to rubbles with just one typhoon.

9. Transport

Your Porsche will end up useless during floods. In several countries, news reports showed people swimming their way to their destination. Some are stuck where they are because there is no available transportation. Strong winds can knock down trees, making roads inaccessible for vehicles.

10. Landscape

The sad thing about what we are doing to nature is how the effects of the damage we did to it will also be experienced by nature. It is not only humans who are going to be affected. When super typhoons come into a country, trees are uprooted as if not enough trees have been cut down by humans. Ecosystems could be reduced into nothing, historical and cultural landscapes could be damaged, and green spaces could be obliterated.

Chapter 6 - Response to Climate Change

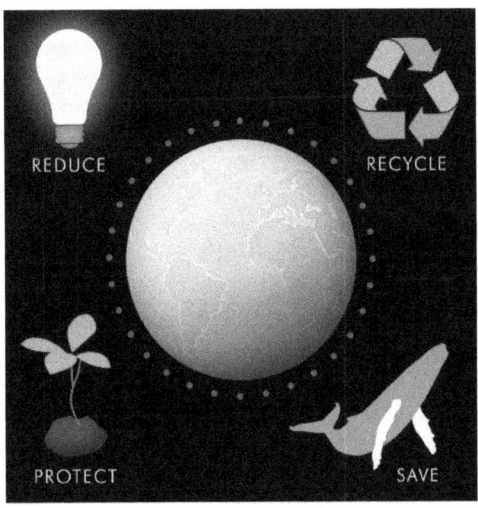

The man-made greenhouse gases that are present in the atmosphere brought about by human activities will continue to have their effects. They will trap solar radiation and warm Earth for the succeeding centuries. In other words, climate change could be inevitable given the severity of our environmental state and people would then have to be forced to adapt to a world with rising temperature. What the future will look like, whether it becomes an inhospitable world full of calamities or one with relatively moderate change in climate, depends on how far we can curtail human activities that are changing the planet. As decision-makers, we have a say which of the two scenarios we would like.

There are a lot of things we can do. Just because it is a given that we would be facing some of the effects of climate change in the years to come does not mean our hands are tied. In fact, the execution of certain actions are still necessary in order to stabilize the concentrations of greenhouse gases in the atmosphere. One of the objectives that would greatly help is to stop the concentration of GHG from increasing altogether. Global emission of GHG must decline – and ideally stop – in the next decades.

Climate Change

In general, there are two ways to respond to climate change: mitigate and adapt. Mitigation refers to the formulation and implementation of regulations and interventions aimed to reduce the concentration of greenhouse gases in the atmosphere and invest on methods that could remove them such as vegetation and forests.

Currently, there is an international mechanism that pushes countries into reducing the quantity of their emissions and that is the UNFCCC or United Nations Framework Convention on Climate Change. The UNFCCC is a treaty whose goal is to stabilize GHG concentrations in the atmosphere. It provided a framework for protocols to the participating countries. Through it, the Kyoto Protocol, which instituted legally binding obligations for the countries involved to reduce their GHG emissions, was developed. The task now for countries is to make soundproof and enforceable policies that will limit the GHG emissions of their constituents. For large, developed countries like the U.S. who happens to be responsible for half of the man-made emissions in the atmosphere, there is an additional duty of being a role model for other countries to follow. It is about time that environmental issues come to the fore. Status quo presents the economy as the number one priority of institutions with problems pertaining to nature taking a backseat.

As an individual, there are a lot of things you can do to mitigate the progress of climate change and take part in not furthering the destruction of our planet. Whether at home or in the office, every major moves you make can affect the state of our Earth and you should therefore think twice about your daily activities.

1. Travel smart.

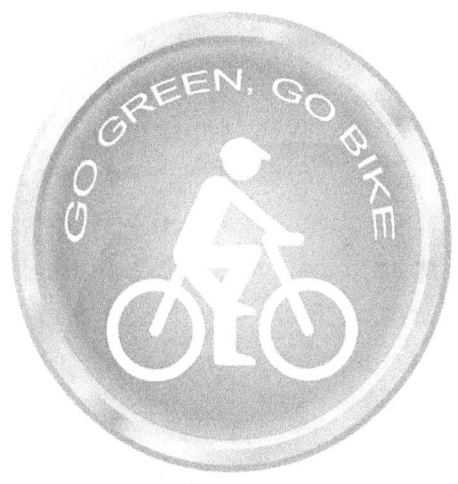

If there is a need to purchase a car, choose one that causes as less damage as possible. There are already green cars available in the market that does not need gas to run. You can also go over cars with high-mileage like hybrids and plug-in hybrids since they use relatively less gas. This way, you can also save money. Think before you buy. Ask and compare fuel economy performance before you make your final decision.

If, in all honesty, you have the chance to not use a car, choose better modes of transportation. Remember that the transport section is the greatest contributor of CO_2 emissions in the air. Perhaps you can bike or walk instead towards your destination. To save gas, take the public transit more and perform your errands in one session so you do not have to continuously travel.

Choosing to live in a community that encourages less driving can also help. If your place of residence depends on your workplace, find one that is close so you can afford just walking to and from work.

2. Be energy-efficient.

The world will benefit if we get smarter in our dealings with energy. Case in point, using more effective and efficient methods in heating, cooling, insulating, and lighting in our buildings can greatly reduce GHG emissions. If there is really a demand to procure home appliances, choose those that are energy-efficient as well.

Avoid using incandescent bulbs. Go for compact fluorescent bulbs instead since they will last ten times longer. Compact fluorescent bulbs also emit lesser CO_2 into the atmosphere and have a lower corresponding energy bill.

The tip when buying new products is to look for the EPA's energy star label to guide you in making the best decision. There are now a lot of products, from lighting productions to electronic gadgets, out there with the energy star label.

3. Use water efficiently.

Energy is consumed in extracting water from its source, treating, and heating it so you can use it for drinking, bating, etc.

Meaning, saving water would lessen emissions of greenhouse gases. In your home, saving water is easily done. As much as possible, lessen the amount of water that you consume and do not waste it. For one, avoid letting the water run as you brush your teeth. In taking showers, limit your time in the bathroom. Some people, instead of using the showers, bathe from water containers and pails instead so they can control the amount of water that they use. This way, you do not excessively consume water.

In washing your dishes, wait for a full load and save dirty water for purposes such as flushing the toilet.

4. Reduce carbon footprint

A very good method in helping curb the hastening pace of climate change is to reduce one's carbon footprint. Meaning, you emit as less GHG as you can. In today's world, this is very difficult to achieve since we are so dependent on technology that runs on fuel. An extreme solution would be to go back to a minimalist lifestyle akin to cavepeople but admittedly, that would be hard to achieve. However, no one is stopping us from starting it small. We can engage in the most common way in reducing carbon footprint and that is to reduce, reuse, recycle, and refuse.

Recycling and reusing helps a lot because in the process of extracting the raw materials for the product, manufacturing and distributing it to the consumers, and disposing it, greenhouse gases are emitted. You can reduce GHG emissions if manufacturers do not have to always make new products. The 4R would also help curb the problem of pollution in the planet.

Engage in recycling programs in your community and if there is not one, think about taking the initiative of starting one. Also, compost your food and other biodegradables to reduce the amount of garbage that goes into landfills.

5. Practice environmentally-friendly habits wherever you are.

Whether you are at home or at work, engage in behavior that would benefit the environment. Some of the important things you can do is to turn off your appliances when they are not in use. Do not let them stay idle. Your computer, for example, should be shut down instead of just being logged off after you are using it.

Make an effort to make your space green. At home, if you do not have space for a garden, you can purchase pots or make use of plastic bottles and use them for vertical gardening. In your office, bring in plants and talk to those in authority to enforce environmental policies.

6. Lessen primary demands for services and goods that would require energy.

Honestly, this is a very difficult feat to achieve since we are so dependent on fuel but it is a step we could take for reduce our carbon footprint. We should learn to sift through our wants and needs. Is getting pampered in the salon for half a day really necessary? Should electricity be in the picture? If you want a massage, you can always have one without burning fuels as you do so. Or if you want to dry your hair, how about letting the natural air do it for you instead of blow drying it?

Institutions, instead of only thinking about gaining profit, should think about incorporating incentive and knowledge programs that would steer consumer preferences and behavior away from choices that would require burning of energy.

7. Encourage the use of low and zero-carbon energy sources

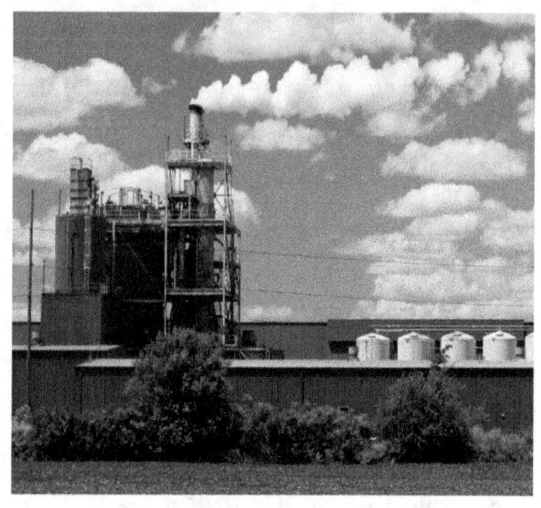

The burning of coals, oils, natural gas, and the utilization of geothermal power, hydroelectricity, nuclear power, wind power, etc., all have carbon footprints. But among these sources of electricity, wind, hydroelectric and nuclear power produced the least amount of carbon dioxide so this is something that countries need to think about.

Switching from oil and coal as energy sources to zero-carbon energy sources such as natural gas will also do a great deal of good. Institutions must also invest in finding alternative sources of fuel and veer away from drawing power from GHG-emitting energy sources. Some countries are already doing this but it would me more ideal if more countries turn to renewable energy sources which include wind, solar, geothermal, biomass, and hydropower.

8. Spread the word.

Make an effort in telling other people and making them aware of the state of our planet. Share with them tips to conserve energy and emphasize how important it is to lower the concentration of greenhouse gases. Even if you manage to convince only two people to adapt an environmentally-friendly lifestyle, that is already a great step towards the mending of our planet.

Another way to respond to climate change would be to adapt to its effects. It involves the engagement in preparation for and minimizing the expected effects of climate change. Adaptation is a process through which human societies equip themselves with the capacity to deal with an uncertain future. To adapt to climate change would mean practicing the right actions in order lessen its negative impacts and take advantage of positive ones if they do exist.

In several states, they are already devising adaptation plans and response mechanisms. However, what they have formulated their plans on are historical records of climate changes which are relatively stable and moderate in nature. However, the climate change of today is quite different and whose effects are more intense. Therefore, there is a need to break away from the perspective of past climate changes and anticipate one that is at its worst. Only in considering a wide range of possible and horrible climate conditions can we consider ourselves close to ready.

For countries who have already framed their adaptation plans, good for them. Yet, what is noteworthy is that there are still countries who are nowhere near prepared. Some of them do not even deem climate change as a pressing issue. For some cases, this is understandable for there are nations who are currently in the middle of conflicts with other nations and they prioritize focusing on immediate threats that they could see. What they need to realize sooner rather than later is that the threat of climate change is not centuries ahead but is looming by a few decades.

So even though there are still questions and ambiguities in terms of the exact intensity, magnitude, and nature of the impacts of climate change, it is vital to mobilize now the constituents of a country. National, regional, and local efforts to inform and prepare the masses must be exerted. People should be made aware and be taught to plan for themselves for worst-case scenarios.

The goal at the end of the day is to guarantee minimal damage and life loss and ensure that there are enough resources left to sustain organic life. In the following section are some examples of adaptation plans and strategies as responses to climate change.

Climate Change

1. Making use of technology

Yes, technology is one of the reasons why we are about to face hell on Earth but we can also turn it into a tool to help us be prepared. We can increase our defenses against the rising sea level by creating sea walls or extending the shoreline or creating flood-proof houses using technology.

2. Changing human behavior

In cases of disasters, human beings should learn to adapt to the situation and learn fast. When it is drought, reduce water consumption, for example. Furthermore, it is important to be more knowledgeable about climate change. Remaining ignorant about it just because you do not feel like it is a serious threat would put your life at risk. Take the graveness of the issue at heart and respond to it properly.

3. Devise early warning systems

Countries and their constituents should invest on proper and effective early warning systems to minimize deaths. If people are made aware beforehand of an incoming disaster, there would be sufficient time for preparation.

4. Improvise disaster risk management

Lives have been lost because of improper risk management plans. A sound plan should be able to address various scenarios and should be detailed enough to cover any issue.

5. Engage in reforestation

This is not only to solve the huge problem of deforestation but also, when located near the coast, could serve as protection against storm surges.

6. Water management

As one of the basic necessities, water is a very important resource and should be properly managed. The impact of climate change can lead to water shortage and contamination so it is an imperative that individuals and countries provide solutions to every possible event that could happen to their water supplies. Conservation of water catchment areas could be encouraged, as an example of anticipatory adaptation strategies, as well as development of flood controls and drought monitoring. Protection and maintenance of existing water supply systems should also be observed.

7. Protect terrestrial ecosystems

People must not neglect the other organisms in this planet as they prepare for any calamity. While institutions are trying their best to preserve human lives, those of animals and plants must also be taken into careful consideration. Some examples of strategies regarding the protection of ecosystems include identification of vulnerable ecosystems, monitoring of plant and animal species, improvement of wildfire management plans, creation of protected areas, etc.

8. Secure food

Measures to ensure that there will be food supplies during and after natural calamities should be met. To respond to changes in weather patterns, farmers could alternate between type of crops and match crops to the weather they are more likely to survive in. Early warning systems intended for agricultural farmlands should also be devised. Farmers could also think about changing their planting and harvesting times as well as diversifying their crops. Research should also be targeted into the development of crops that are resistant to the effects of climate change. Perhaps there can be crops that will be tolerant or even resistant against drought.

9. Look into human health

Institutions must look into what services and situations can best facilitate human mortality. Perhaps changes in housing design is needed to guarantee that in case of floods, houses and the people inside are not swept away. The health sector should also place importance in improving their facilities so they could treat potential victims as best as possible.

10. Awareness campaigns

This is an important adaptation strategy because without knowledge, people would not know what to act on and why. People should be made aware by different government bodies on what to prepare. There should be an active attempt in instilling survival tips and preservation strategies into the minds of people. And while doing so, the urgency of the issue must be made clear.

You, as an individual, do not need to wait for the government or any authority to spoon feed you with information. This book, in fact, is a step towards preparing yourself. What you can further do is make use of technology and learn all that you can about what climate change can do and how it can affect your life and that of the people you love. And do not just stop with acquiring knowledge. Make sure that you are applying what you learn. If you realized how important it is to conserve water, start right at this moment to consume less.

CONCLUSION

Thank you again for downloading this book!

Human activity is ultimately the greatest reason for the instability of the planet and the damages it is incurring right now. No amount of natural variability could explain the pace of which Earth is changing and devolving. From deforestation to technological advancement, human beings have done a lot to damage Earth and exploit its resources whether intentionally or unintentionally. Despite how bleak this situation might be in the coming decades, the positive thing to remember about this is that we have options.

It all boils down to two choices: (a) make no serious effort in combating and alleviating the effects of global warming and other implications of climate change

and just cope with the resulting disasters
Mother Earth throws our way or (b) be
responsible and act now to mitigate
prospective damage to our homes,
communities, and environment. It takes
commitment and hard work to stick with
the second choice but it is the *better*
choice. Governments and organizations
have attempted to make progress already
in fighting against global warming.
Policies, treaties, and laws have been
drafted that are meant to be implemented
at international, national, and local levels
and everyone's task is to think into the
future and dwell on what will happen if
we fail to do the right thing now.

We are unaware of it at times but we have
in our hands the bombs that can destroy
Earth once and for all. But what we must
remember is the fact that along with the
destruction of Earth is our destruction, as
well. So far, this is the only planet that can
support us and it is our responsibility to

take care of it not just for the sake of this generation but also for the succeeding ones.

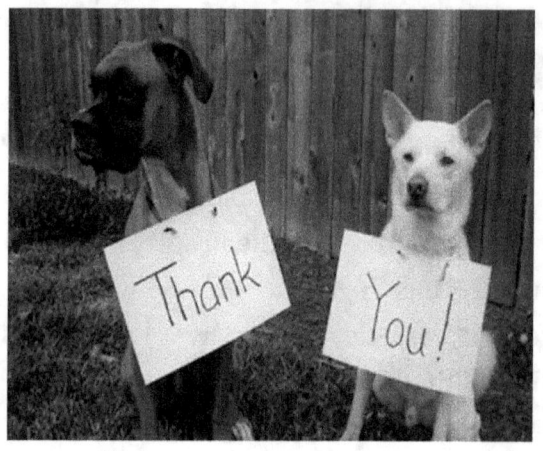

Finally, if you enjoyed this book, then I'd like to ask you for a favor, would you be kind enough to leave a review for this book on Amazon? It'd be greatly appreciated!

Thank you and good luck!

www.ingramcontent.com/pod-product-compliance
Lightning Source LLC
Chambersburg PA
CBHW071223280526
45787CB00002B/775

* 9 7 8 1 5 1 7 4 8 8 0 4 8 *